YOGA FOR SENIORS OVER 50

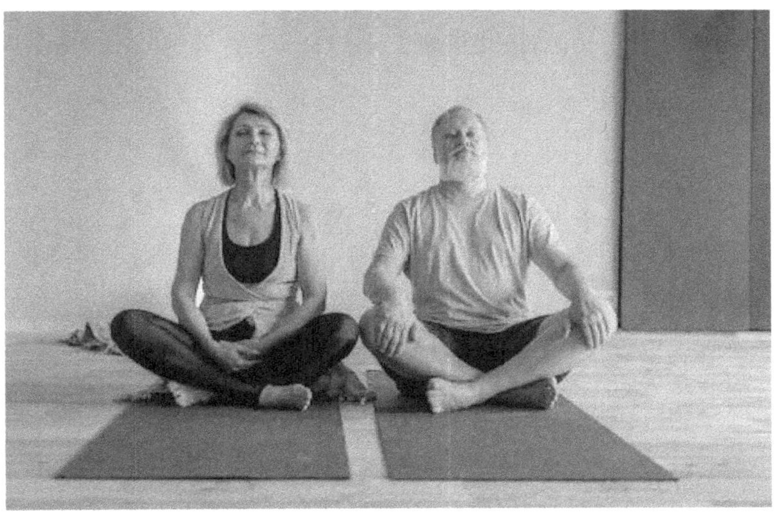

Dr. Kimberly Carlos

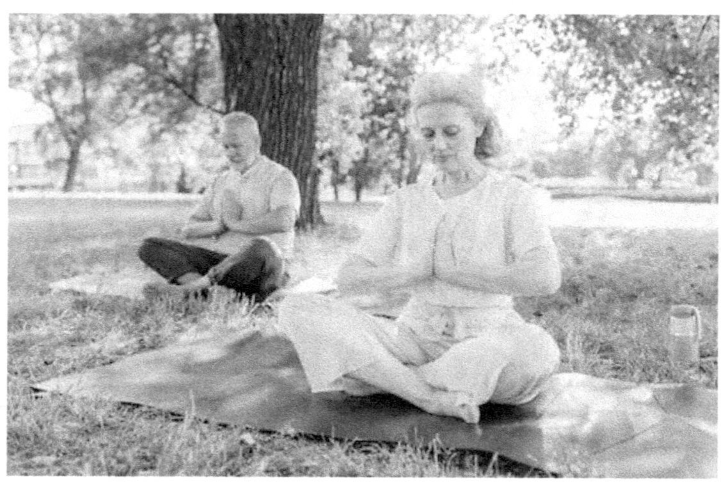

TABLE OF CONTENT

INTRODUCTION

In a quaint little town, nestled among rolling hills and surrounded by a serene landscape, lived an enthusiastic and compassionate soul named Sarah. At 55 years young, Sarah was determined to spread the joy of yoga to her fellow seniors in the community.

After retiring from her successful career as a teacher, Sarah discovered her love for yoga. She realized that yoga not only kept her physically fit but also brought immense peace and mental clarity.

She noticed that many seniors in her town, though eager to experience the benefits of yoga, were hesitant due to their age and physical limitations.

Undeterred, Sarah decided to embark on a mission to introduce yoga to seniors over 50. She gathered her knowledge from years of practicing and attending various workshops, specifically tailoring the practice to accommodate the needs of older individuals.

Every morning, as the sun rose, Sarah would set up her yoga mats in the tranquil park at the heart of the town.

Her infectious smile and warm demeanor attracted seniors from all walks of life. Some were curious newcomers, while others had heard of her reputation and returned regularly.

Sarah began each session with gentle warm-up exercises to ease stiffness and promote flexibility. She emphasized the importance of mindful breathing and encouraged her students to let go of any stress or worries.

As the group moved through different yoga postures, Sarah made sure to offer modifications for those with limited mobility, ensuring everyone felt included and safe.

The seniors quickly realized the benefits of their newfound practice. They felt more energetic, their joints became less achy, and they noticed a positive shift in their overall outlook on life.

But perhaps the most significant impact was the sense of community that blossomed among the participants. Friendships formed, and laughter echoed through the park during and after each session.

Word about Sarah's yoga for seniors over 50 classes spread like wildfire.

Soon, the park couldn't contain the growing number of eager participants. Undeterred, Sarah partnered with the local community center, where she continued her classes indoors during colder months and rainy days.

As the months passed, the group became a close-knit family. They celebrated each other's milestones and provided unwavering support during challenging times. Sarah, delighted to witness the transformation in her students, felt a profound sense of fulfillment in her heart.

One day, a local newspaper featured Sarah's story, highlighting her dedication and the positive impact she had on the lives of so many seniors. The article caught the attention of nearby towns, and requests poured in for Sarah to conduct workshops and classes in their communities too.

Embracing the opportunity, Sarah expanded her reach, and her message of yoga for seniors over 50 touched lives far and wide. She became an inspiration for others to follow their passions and make a difference, regardless of age or circumstance.

And so, the once serene town became a hub of rejuvenation and positivity, all thanks to Sarah's unwavering commitment to bringing the gift of yoga to those who needed it the most. As the sun set each day, casting a golden glow over the park where it all began, Sarah's heart swelled with gratitude for the beautiful journey she had embarked upon.

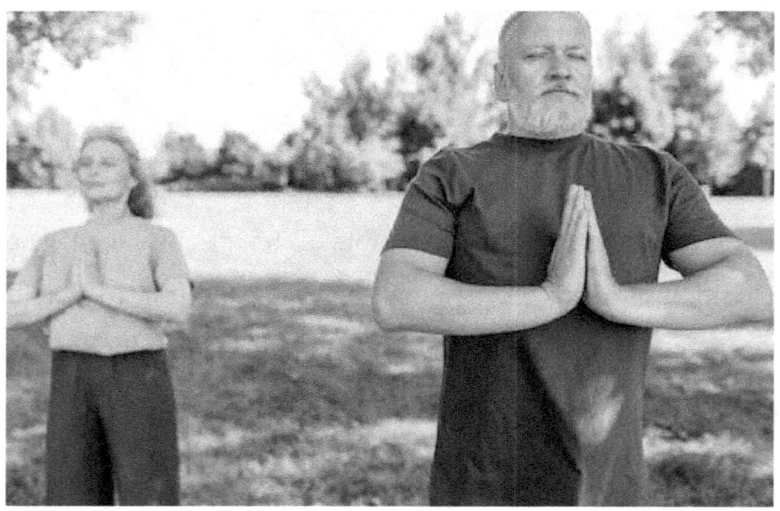

CHAPTER ONE

Yoga for Seniors Benefits

Aging is a natural process that brings with it wisdom and experience, but it can also present certain challenges, both physically and mentally. As we grow older, it becomes essential to prioritize our health and well-being.

One fantastic way to achieve this is through the practice of yoga for seniors. Yoga offers a holistic approach to maintaining physical strength, flexibility, mental clarity, and emotional balance.

The Unique Benefits of Yoga for Seniors

1. Improved Flexibility and Mobility: With age, our joints may become stiffer, and muscles might lose their elasticity. Yoga involves gentle stretches and poses that target these areas, promoting increased flexibility and range of motion.

2. Enhanced Balance and Stability: Yoga poses often require focus and concentration, which can significantly improve balance and stability. For seniors at risk of falls, this aspect of yoga can be particularly beneficial in preventing accidents and injuries.

3. Stress Relief and Relaxation: Seniors often face life changes, including retirement, loss of loved ones, or health issues. Yoga incorporates relaxation techniques, deep breathing, and meditation, reducing stress and promoting a sense of calm and tranquility.

4. Pain Management: Many older individuals experience chronic pain conditions such as arthritis or back pain. Certain yoga poses and movements can help alleviate pain and discomfort by gently stretching and strengthening the affected areas.

5. Increased Mindfulness: Mindfulness is the art of being present and fully aware of one's thoughts and emotions. Through yoga, seniors can cultivate mindfulness, enhancing their ability to cope with challenges and embrace the present moment.

6. Heart Health: Some forms of yoga involve gentle cardiovascular exercises, which can help improve heart health and circulation. As heart-related issues become more prevalent with age, maintaining a healthy heart is of utmost importance.

7. Community and Social Interaction: Attending yoga classes for seniors provides an opportunity to meet like-minded individuals and build a supportive community. Social interaction is crucial for mental well-being and can combat feelings of loneliness or isolation.

How to Start a Yoga Practice as a Senior

Starting a yoga practice as a senior is an exciting journey, but it's essential to approach it with patience and an open mind. To get you started, follow these steps:

1. Consult with Your Doctor: Before beginning any new exercise regimen, it's crucial to consult with your healthcare provider, especially if you have any pre-existing medical conditions or concerns.

2. Find a Suitable Class: Look for yoga classes specifically designed for seniors or beginners. These classes often focus on gentle movements and provide modifications for various fitness levels and abilities.

3. Invest in Proper Equipment: A good-quality yoga mat, comfortable clothing, and some props like blocks and straps can enhance your practice and make it more enjoyable.

4. Start Slowly: It's okay to take your time and ease into the practice. Consider your body's limitations and pay attention to them. Keep in mind that yoga is a personal path of self-discovery, not a sport.

5. Practice Mindful Breathing: Breathwork is an integral part of yoga. Learn to practice deep, mindful breathing as it helps calm the mind and relax the body.

6. Be Consistent: Regularity is key to experiencing the full benefits of yoga. Try to incorporate short yoga sessions into your daily routine and gradually increase the duration as you become more comfortable.

7. Be Kind to Yourself: Don't be discouraged by any initial challenges or limitations. Yoga is a non-judgmental practice, and every individual progresses at their own pace.

Safe and Beneficial Poses for Seniors

Here are some gentle yoga poses that can be particularly beneficial for seniors:

1. Mountain Pose (Tadasana): This standing pose promotes alignment, improves posture, and enhances body awareness.

2. Cat-Cow Stretch: A gentle flow between these two poses helps to lubricate the spine and improves flexibility.

3. Child's Pose (Balasana): A resting pose that stretches the back and promotes relaxation.

4. Bridge Pose (Setu Bandha Sarvangasana): Strengthens the legs and back while opening the chest and shoulders.

5. Legs Up the Wall (Viparita Karani): A restorative pose that helps reduce swelling in the legs and promotes relaxation.

6. Tree Pose (Vrikshasana): Enhances balance and focus while stretching the hips and legs.

7. Corpse Pose (Savasana): The final relaxation pose that allows the body and mind to fully relax and integrate the benefits of the practice.

Incorporate Mindfulness and Meditation

Yoga for seniors goes beyond physical postures; it also includes mindfulness and meditation. These practices can further improve mental well-being and provide clarity and peace. Consider adding a short meditation session to your daily routine, focusing on your breath or using guided meditation apps or videos.

Yoga for seniors is a beautiful and gentle way to stay active, maintain mental clarity, and nurture a sense of well-being as we age gracefully. Embrace this ancient practice with an open heart, and you'll discover the transformative benefits it offers for your body, mind, and soul.

Remember that yoga is not about perfection; it's about progress and the journey towards finding harmony within yourself. Embrace the practice, and you'll find yourself reaping its numerous rewards in all aspects of your life. Namaste!

CHAPTER TWO

14 Day Yoga for Seniors Over 50 Meal Plan

Maintaining a healthy and balanced diet is essential for seniors practicing yoga. A well-rounded meal plan can provide the necessary nutrients to support their practice and overall well-being.

This comprehensive 14-day meal plan is designed specifically for seniors over 50 who engage in yoga, focusing on nourishing foods that promote energy, flexibility, and mental clarity.

DAY 1

- Breakfast: Greek yogurt topped with mixed berries and a sprinkle of nuts.
- Lunch: Quinoa and roasted vegetable salad with a lemon-tahini dressing.
- Dinner: Baked salmon with steamed broccoli and sweet potato.

DAY 2

- Breakfast: spinach, banana, almond milk, and chia seed smoothie.
- Lunch: Lentil soup with a side of mixed greens and a whole-grain roll.
- Dinner: Grilled chicken breast with asparagus and brown rice.

DAY 3

- Breakfast: Oatmeal topped with sliced peaches, a drizzle of honey, and chopped walnuts.
- Lunch: Chickpea and cucumber salad with feta cheese and a lemon-herb dressing.
- Dinner: Stir-fried tofu with mixed vegetables and Quinoa.

Day 4

- Breakfast: Whole-grain toast with avocado and poached eggs.
- Lunch: Spinach and feta stuffed chicken breast with a side of roasted Brussels sprouts.
- Dinner: Baked cod with a side of sautéed spinach and quinoa.

DAY 5

- Breakfast: Cottage cheese with sliced peaches and a sprinkle of sunflower seeds.
- Lunch: Vegetable and bean chili with a side of cornbread.
- Dinner: Grilled shrimp skewers with roasted sweet potatoes and green beans.

DAY 6

- Breakfast: Smoothie with mixed berries, banana, Greek yogurt, and flaxseed.
- Lunch: Spinach and mushroom frittata with a side of mixed greens.
- Dinner: Baked chicken thighs with roasted carrots and wild rice.

DAY 7

- Breakfast: Chia seed pudding topped with mango and coconut flakes.
- Lunch: Quinoa and black bean salad with avocado and a lime-cilantro dressing.
- Dinner: Stuffed bell peppers with lean ground turkey and a side of steamed broccoli.

DAY 8

Breakfast: Whole-grain waffles topped with fresh berries and a dollop of Greek yogurt.

Lunch: Lentil and vegetable stir-fry with a side of brown rice.

Dinner: Grilled salmon with sautéed kale and sweet potato wedges.

DAY 9

- Breakfast: Scrambled eggs with spinach and tomatoes, served with whole-grain toast.
- Lunch: Chickpea and quinoa bowl with roasted vegetables and a lemon-tahini dressing.
- Dinner: Baked tilapia with a side of steamed asparagus and couscous.

DAY 10

- Breakfast: Smoothie with kale, pineapple, banana, and almond milk.
- Lunch: Spinach and feta stuffed portobello mushrooms with a side of mixed greens.
- Dinner: Baked chicken breast with roasted Brussels sprouts and sweet potato mash.

DAY 11

- Breakfast: Yogurt parfait with granola, mixed berries, and a drizzle of honey.
- Lunch: Vegetable and lentil soup served with whole-grain crackers on the side.
- Dinner: Grilled shrimp with a quinoa and vegetable medley.

DAY 12

- Breakfast: Overnight oats with almond milk, sliced apples, and a sprinkle of cinnamon.
- Lunch: Chickpea salad with cucumber, bell peppers, and a lemon-herb dressing.
- Dinner: Baked cod with roasted broccoli and wild rice.

DAY 13

- Breakfast: Whole-grain toast with almond butter and sliced banana.
- Lunch: Vegetable and tofu stir-fry with a side of brown rice.
- Dinner: Grilled chicken skewers with zucchini noodles and tomato sauce.

DAY 14

- Breakfast: Scrambled eggs with diced tomatoes and spinach, served with a whole-grain English muffin.
- Lunch: Quinoa and vegetable stuffed bell peppers with a side of mixed greens.
- Dinner: Baked salmon with steamed asparagus and couscous.

Snack Options (choose 1-2 daily)

- Mixed nuts and seeds.
- Fresh fruit (e.g., apple slices with almond butter).
- Veggie sticks with hummus.
- Greek yogurt with honey and granola.
- Rice cakes with cherry tomatoes and avocado.

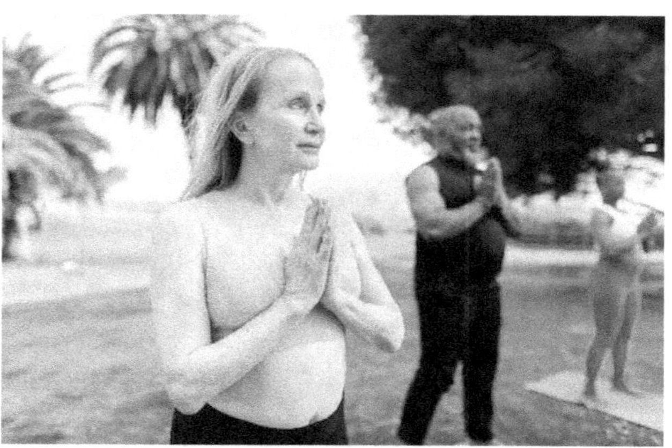

CHAPTER THREE

40 Yoga for Seniors Over 50 Exercises and How to Do Them

1. Mountain Pose (Tadasana)

- Stand tall with feet hip-width apart.

- Lengthen your spine and relax your shoulders.

- Gently engage your core and breathe deeply.

2. Cat-Cow Stretch

- Get into a tabletop position and start off on your hands and knees.

- As you breathe in, arch your back and elevate your head in the "Cow Pose."

- Exhale, round your back, and tuck your chin (Cat Pose).

- Repeat in a gentle flowing motion.

3. Child's Pose (Balasana)

- Get on all fours and bend over, kneeling.
- As you lower your chest to the floor, extend your arms in front of you.
- Breathe deeply as you place your forehead down on the mat.

4. Downward Facing Dog (Adho Mukha Svanasana)

- From tabletop position, tuck your toes, lift your hips, and straighten your legs.
- Extend your fingers widely and firmly plant your palms on the ground.
- Tighten your abs while letting your neck down.

5. Standing Forward Bend (Uttanasana)

- Stand with feet hip-width apart.
- Hinge at your hips and fold forward, reaching towards the floor.
- Bend your knees slightly if needed to keep your spine straight.

6. Seated Forward Bend (Paschimottanasana)

- Place your legs out in front of you when you sit.
- Lengthen your spine as you inhale, and then bend forward at the hips as you exhale.
- Reach for your ankles, shins, or toes.

7. Warrior II (Virabhadrasana II)

- Place your feet wider than shoulder-width apart and extend your right foot.
- Keeping your left leg straight, bend your right knee to a 90-degree angle.
- Look over your right hand while spreading your arms out to the sides.

8. Warrior I (Virabhadrasana I)

- From Warrior II, pivot your back foot slightly inward.
- Square your hips and lift your arms overhead, palms facing each other.

9. Triangle Pose (Trikonasana)

- Stand with feet wide apart, turn your right foot outward.
- Reach your right arm forward, hinge at your hip, and lower your right hand to your shin.
- Raise your left arm toward the sky.

10. Bridge Pose (Setu Bandha Sarvangasana)

- Lie on your back with your feet flat on the ground and your knees bent.
- Press your feet into the ground and lift your hips, creating a bridge shape.
- Interlace your fingers under your back for support.

11. Tree Pose (Vrikshasana)

- Stand with feet hip-width apart and shift your weight to your left foot.
- Place your right foot on your left ankle, calf, or thigh (avoid the knee).
- Join your hands at the location of your heart.

12. Cobra Pose (Bhujangasana)

- Lie on your stomach with palms beside your shoulders.
- Take a breath, squeeze your hands together, and raise your chest off the ground.
- Relax your shoulders and keep your elbows close to your body.

13. Extended Triangle Pose (Utthita Trikonasana)

- Stand with feet wide apart, turn your right foot outward.
- Reach your right arm forward and hinge at your hip to lower your right hand to your shin.
- Raise your left arm toward the sky.

14. Shoulder Rolls

- Maintain a straight back while you stand or sit.
- Breathe in and raise your shoulders to your ears.
- Exhale, roll them back and down.

15. Neck Stretches

- Sit tall and gently tilt your head to the right, feeling a stretch along the left side of your neck.
- Repeat on the left side.
- Chin should be lowered to chest level and then raised to the ceiling.

16. Seated Spinal Twist

- Place your legs out in front of you when you sit.

- Cross your right foot over your left knee and place your right hand behind you.

- Inhale, lengthen your spine, and exhale, twist to the right, placing your left elbow outside your right knee.

17. Half Lord of the Fishes (Ardha Matsyendrasana)

- Sit with legs extended, bend your right knee and place your right foot outside your left thigh.

- Inhale, lift your left arm, and exhale, twist to the right, hooking your left elbow outside your right knee.

18. Seated Forward Bend with a Strap

- Sit tall with legs extended and place a strap around the balls of your feet.

- Inhale, lengthen your spine, and exhale, hinge forward at your hips, holding the strap.

19. Supported Bridge Pose

- Lie on your back with your feet flat on the ground and your knees bent.
- Place your hips on a block or pillow that you've slid beneath your sacrum.
- Breathe deeply while you relax your arms at your sides.

20. Wide-Legged Forward Bend (Prasarita Padottanasana)

- Stand with feet wide apart and hinge at your hips, folding forward.
- Place your hands on the floor or a block for support.
- Keep your spine long and your legs engaged.

21. Seated Twist with Legs Crossed

- Sit with legs crossed and your right hand on your left knee.
- Inhale, lengthen your spine, and exhale, twist to the left.
- Gaze over your left shoulder.

22. Reclining Bound Angle Pose (Supta Baddha Konasana)

- Lie on your back with your feet together and your knees bent.
- Spread your knees out to the sides, forming the shape of a diamond with your legs.
- Put your arms at your sides in a relaxed position.

23. Cow Face Pose (Gomukhasana) Arms

- Stand tall and cross your legs in front of you.
- Reach behind you with your right elbow bent.
- Reach your left arm up and bend it to reach towards your right hand.

24. Supported Shoulderstand with a Wall

- Lie on your back with your hips close to a wall.
- Lift your legs up the wall, supporting your lower back with your hands.
- Keep your legs straight and breathe deeply.

25. Seated Side Bend

-   Sit tall with legs extended to the right side.

-   Inhale, reach your left arm up and exhale, bend to the right side.

-   Avoid collapsing on your right side; maintain length in your spine.

26. Garland Pose (Malasana)

-   Stand with feet wider than hip-width apart and toes slightly turned outward.

-   Squat down by bending your knees and bringing your hips down.

-   At the location of your heart, converge your palms.

27. Butterfly Pose (Baddha Konasana)

-   Sit tall with the soles of your feet touching each other.

-   Keep your spine straight and take a deep breath.

-   Hold your feet with your hands and softly press your knees toward the floor.

28. Corpse Pose (Savasana)

- Lie flat on your back with your arms by your sides and your legs outstretched.
- Shut your eyes and concentrate on breathing.
- Allow your body to relax completely.

29. Easy Pose (Sukhasana)

- Cross your legs and sit on the ground or a cushion.
- Place your hands on your lap or knees for support.
- Maintain a straight spine and take deep breaths.

30. Happy Baby Pose (Ananda Balasana)

- Lie on your back and draw your knees towards your chest.
- Hold the outside edges of your feet and gently open your knees wide.
- Relax your shoulders and breathe deeply.

31. Eagle Arms (Garudasana Arms)

- Sit or stand tall and reach your arms forward.
- Cross your right arm over your left, bringing your palms to touch.
- Lift your elbows to shoulder height and breathe deeply.

32. Supported Child's Pose

- Stack several cushions or a bolster in front of you.

- Sit back on your heels and rest your torso on the cushions.

- Extend your arms forward and relax.

33. Supported Fish Pose (Matsyasana)

- Place a block or cushion horizontally behind you.

- Lie on your back with the block supporting your upper back.

- Rest your head back and relax your arms.

34. Supported Legs Up the Wall Pose (Viparita Karani)

- Sit close to a wall with your legs extended upward, resting on the wall.

- Place a cushion under your hips for support.

- Relax your arms by your sides.

35. Supported Wide-Legged Forward Bend

- Sit with legs wide apart and a cushion or block in front of you.

- Hinge at your hips and fold forward, resting your torso on the cushion.

- Relax your arms and breathe deeply.

36. Seated Meditation

- Sit comfortably with your legs crossed or on a cushion.

- Place your hands on your lap or knees for support.

- Shut your eyes and concentrate on breathing.

37. Cow-Face Pose (Gomukhasana) Legs

- Sit upright with your legs out in front of you.

- Stack your knees by crossing your right knee over your left.

- Gently lower your knees to the ground.

38. Sphinx Pose

- Forearms should be on the ground when you lay on your stomach.
- Lift your chest and head off the mat, keeping your elbows under your shoulders.
- Relax your shoulders and breathe deeply.

39. Extended Puppy Pose (Uttana Shishosana)

- Begin in a tabletop position.
- Walk your hands forward, lowering your chest towards the floor.
- Maintain a straight line between your hips and knees.

40. Legs on a Chair Pose

- Sit with your back against a wall and place your legs up on a chair or ottoman.
- Rest your arms comfortably by your sides.
- Relax and breathe deeply.

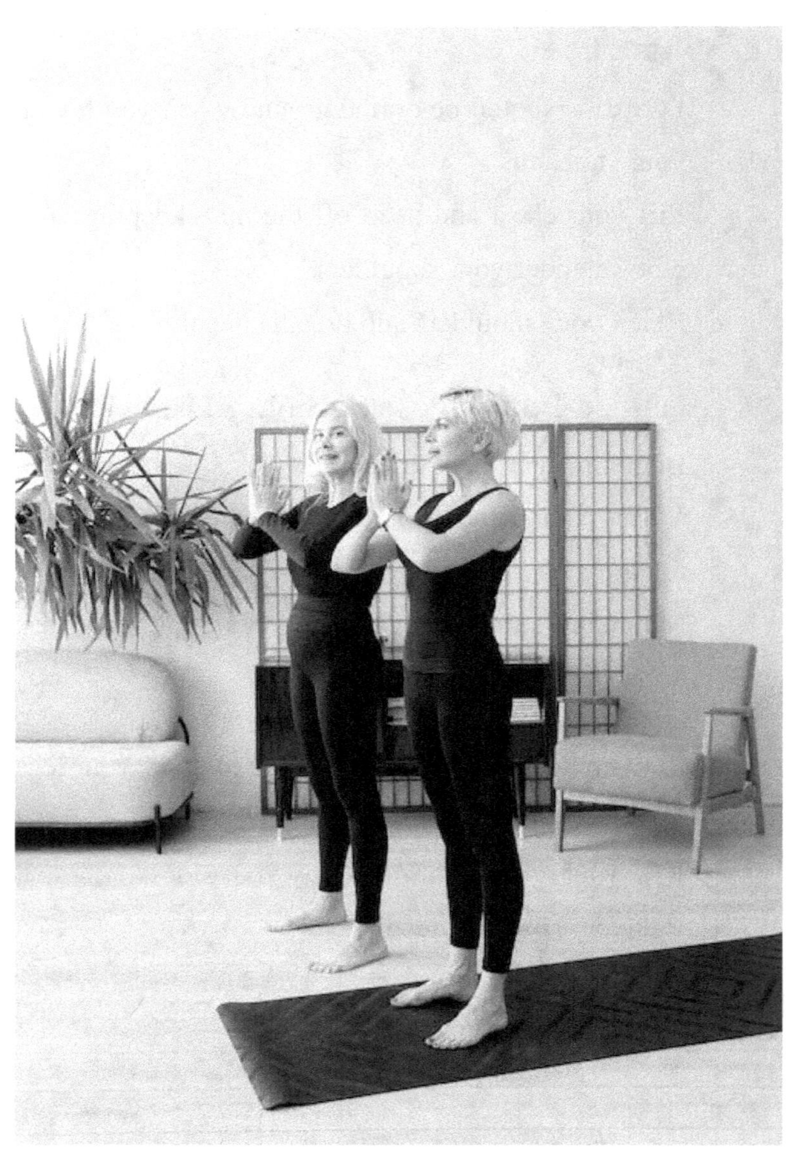

CONCLUSION

Yoga for seniors over 50 is not just a physical practice; it is a transformative journey that touches the mind, body, and soul. As the years go by, it becomes increasingly important to prioritize our health and well-being, and yoga offers a holistic approach to achieve this goal.

Throughout this age group, yoga has proven to be an effective and accessible tool, providing numerous physical, mental, and emotional benefits that contribute to a fulfilling and vibrant life.

Physical Benefits:

For seniors over 50, maintaining flexibility, balance, and strength becomes crucial in promoting mobility and preventing injuries. Yoga's gentle postures and movements offer an ideal way to achieve these goals without putting undue strain on the body.

As participants progress in their practice, they experience increased joint mobility, enhanced muscle tone, and improved posture.

The incorporation of breathwork in yoga helps seniors deepen their lung capacity and oxygen intake, which is especially beneficial for overall respiratory health.

Mental Clarity and Emotional Well-being:

Yoga for seniors over 50 not only nurtures the physical aspect but also brings peace and harmony to the mind. Mindfulness and meditation practices, integral to yoga, enable individuals to become more present and attuned to their thoughts and emotions.

Seniors often experience life transitions, such as retirement or loss of loved ones, which may lead to stress and anxiety. Yoga teaches them to embrace the present moment and find solace amidst life's changes. The relaxation techniques in yoga, like Savasana (Corpse Pose), provide a moment of rest and rejuvenation, alleviating mental fatigue and promoting emotional well-being.

Social Connection and Community:

Attending yoga classes for seniors offers an opportunity to build a supportive community and develop social connections.

Seniors may find themselves at risk of loneliness or isolation, especially after retirement. The welcoming and inclusive atmosphere of yoga classes fosters camaraderie among participants, helping them form meaningful friendships and support systems.

The shared journey of yoga creates a sense of belonging and unity, enriching the lives of individuals within the group.

Personal Growth and Self-Awareness:

As seniors delve into their yoga practice, they embark on a journey of self-discovery and personal growth. Yoga encourages self-awareness, leading to better understanding of one's physical limitations, emotions, and thought patterns. With this heightened self-awareness, seniors can adapt their practice to suit their individual needs and find acceptance in the present moment.

Through yoga, they learn to let go of self-judgment and embrace their unique strengths and vulnerabilities, cultivating a positive self-image and self-confidence.

Empowerment and Independence:

Yoga empowers seniors to take charge of their health and well-being, instilling a sense of autonomy and independence. The gentle nature of yoga allows them to practice at their own pace and make modifications based on their abilities. The knowledge that they can participate in an activity that promotes strength, balance, and mindfulness can boost their confidence and sense of agency.

A Lifelong Journey:

Yoga for seniors over 50 is not a destination; it is a lifelong journey that continues to evolve and unfold with each practice. As seniors develop their practice, they become more attuned to their bodies and minds, allowing them to adapt their practice to meet their changing needs and circumstances. The beauty of yoga lies in its adaptability, making it accessible to individuals of all ages and physical conditions.

In conclusion, yoga for seniors over 50 is a gift that keeps on giving. It offers a sanctuary for the mind, body, and soul, fostering physical well-being, mental clarity, and emotional balance.

The practice of yoga allows seniors to embrace the beauty of aging gracefully, cultivating a deeper sense of self-awareness and self-compassion. Through the camaraderie of a supportive community, seniors discover the joy of shared experiences and a renewed sense of connection.

Yoga is a timeless practice that empowers seniors to embrace life with enthusiasm and vitality, illuminating their path with every breath and asana.

As they continue on their journey, they will find that yoga becomes not just a practice, but a way of life—a transformative and enriching journey of self-discovery and growth. Namaste.

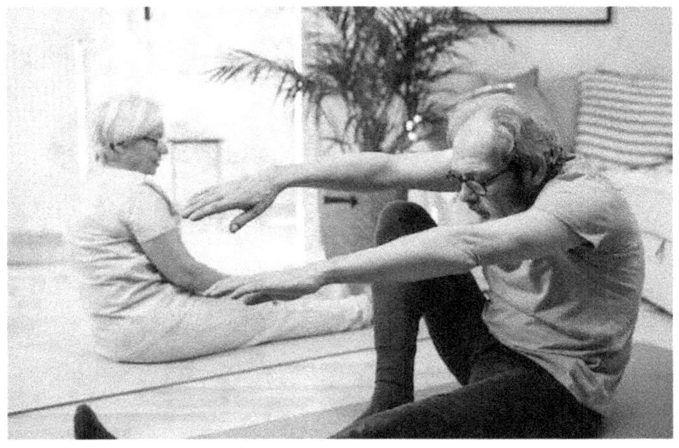

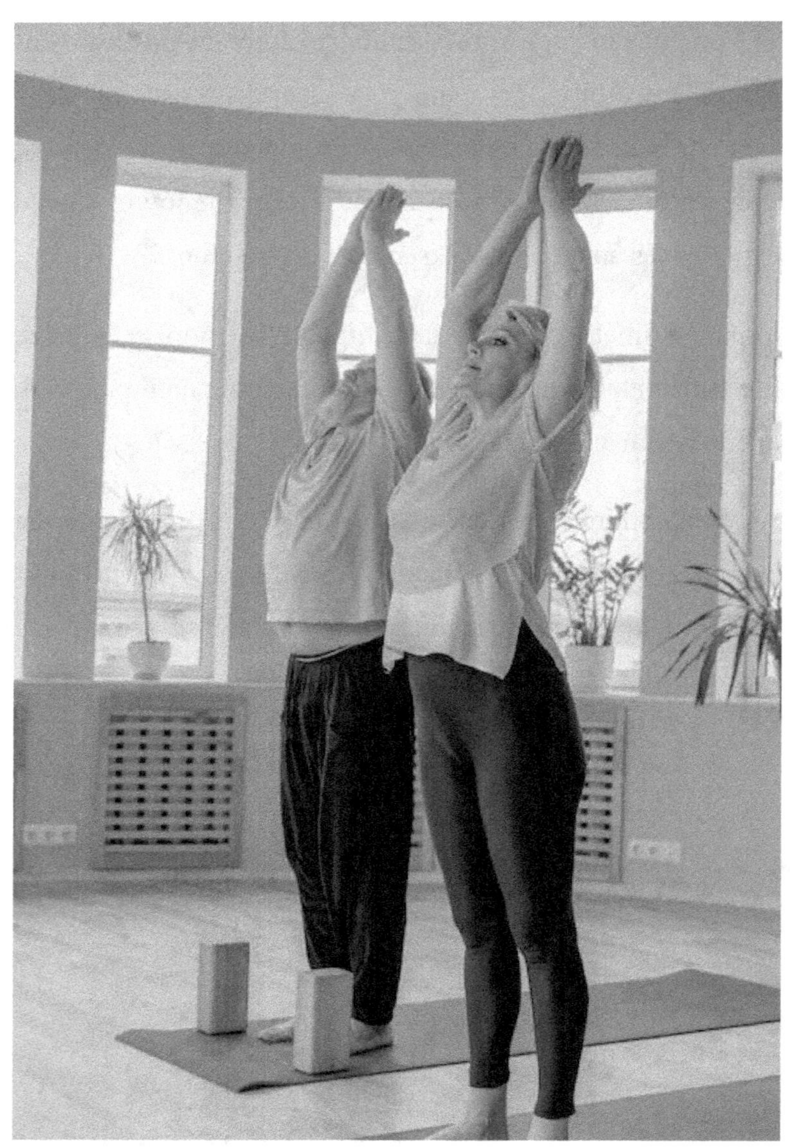